VERTIGO

UNDERSTANDING PERFECTLY HOW VERTIGO WORKS

DR. J. WALLER

Contents

INTRODUCTION

Vertigo is a spinning or dizzying sensation that is commonly characterized as the impression that things are moving around you or that you are moving when they are not. It is a sign of an underlying problem, usually involving the inner ear or the central nervous system, rather than a standalone ailment. A person's balance and coordination can be affected by vertigo, which can range in severity from moderate and transient to severe and ongoing.

Important details regarding vertigo include:

Causes: A number of things can cause vertigo, such as migraines, some drugs, head injuries, brain abnormalities, and inner ear conditions including Meniere's disease or benign paroxysmal positional vertigo.

Symptoms: The spinning or swaying feeling is the main sign of vertigo. Additional symptoms that may be present include sweating, nausea, vomiting, and balance issues.

Vertigo Types:

The cause of peripheral vertigo is problems in the inner ear.

Central vertigo: Associated with issues with the brain and central nervous system.

Diagnosis: Medical professionals employ a variety of methods, including a patient's medical history, a physical examination, and occasionally imaging tests like CT or MRI scans, to determine the cause of vertigo.

The course of treatment for vertigo is determined by its underlying etiology. It could involve taking certain drugs, doing physical therapy exercises, altering one's lifestyle, or having certain inner ear problems treated.

Effect on regular Life: People who experience severe or frequent episodes of vertigo may find it difficult to carry out regular activities including driving, working, or simply walking.

Prevention: Reducing risk factors, controlling stress, and embracing a healthy lifestyle are a few examples of preventive actions.

People who are suffering vertigo should contact a doctor in order to have a proper diagnosis and appropriate treatment. Even while vertigo is not a sickness in and of itself, identifying and treating its underlying causes can assist enhance quality of life and lessen the burden of the condition on day-to-day activities.

CHAPTER ONE

Reasons and Initiators

There are many things that might cause vertigo, but problems with the inner ear or central nervous system are frequently the root reasons. The following are typical vertigo causes and triggers:

Positional vertigo that is benign paroxysmal (BPPV):

One of the most frequent causes of vertigo is BPPV, which happens when tiny calcium crystals in the inner ear fall out of place and enter the ear canals, impairing normal fluid flow.

Meniere's illness:

Meniere's disease is an inner ear ailment that is characterized by vertigo episodes, hearing loss, tinnitus (ear ringing), and an ear fullness sensation.

Diabetic Neuritis:

An inflammation of the vestibular nerve, known as vestibular neuritis, is frequently brought on by viral infections. It causes abrupt vertigo and may also cause instability and nausea.

Headaches:

Vertigo is a symptom that some people get with migraines. Particularly with vestibular migraines, vertigo episodes can accompany headache and other migraine symptoms.

Labyrinthitis:

Inflammation of the inner ear caused by bacteria or viruses is known as labyrinthitis. It may result in ringing in the ears, vertigo, and hearing loss.

Head Injury:

Vertigo can result from traumatic head injuries including concussions that harm the central nervous system or the inner ear.

Drugs:

Vertigo is a side effect of some drugs, especially those that impact the central nervous system or inner ear.

Alterations in blood flow

Vertigo can be brought on by inadequate blood supply to the brain, which is frequently caused by disorders such as orthostatic hypotension or vertebrobasilar insufficiency.

Growths:

Vertigo can be brought on by tumors that impact the vestibular nerve or other CNS components.

Dehydration and Hypoglycemia

Low blood sugar and dehydration both increase the risk of vertigo and dizziness.

Specific Tasks:

In those who are sensitive, head motions, sudden movements, or certain actions like looking up or swiftly twisting the head might cause vertigo.

It's crucial to remember that specific circumstances may differ and that these explanations are not all-inclusive. A medical professional's diagnosis is essential to pinpoint the precise cause of vertigo and choose the best course of action for treatment or management.

Signs and symptoms

In addition to the dizziness or spinning sensation that is its hallmark, vertigo frequently manifests with other symptoms that range in intensity. Typical vertigo symptoms include:

Revolving Sensation:

The main symptom is an illusion of rotational movement, giving the impression that you or your environment are tilting, swaying, or spinning.

Emesis:

Numerous people who have vertigo also have nausea, which can be accompanied by queasiness or an upset stomach.

Throwing up:

Vomiting can occur during severe vertigo episodes, particularly if the feeling is strong and lasts for a long time.

Unstable or Off-balance:

Because vertigo frequently impairs balance and coordination, it can be challenging to walk or stand without support.

Headache:

Headaches can happen to certain persons, especially if vertigo is accompanied by migraines or other underlying medical issues.

Perspiration:

A common sign of vertigo episodes is increased sweating, which is frequently the body's reaction to stress.

Tinnitus or ringing in the ears:

People who have vertigo sometimes also suffer tinnitus, which is a buzzing, ringing, or hissing sound in the ears.

Loss of Hearing:

Hearing loss, either permanent or transient, may accompany vertigo linked to illnesses such as Meniere's disease.

Visual Disturbances:

Episodes of vertigo may cause changes in vision, such as fuzzy vision or trouble focusing.

Nystagmus, or jerking eye movements:

Vertigo may be accompanied with jerky, uncontrollable eye movements (nystagmus), which can be seen by others.

Velocity Sensitivity:

Some people may have an increase in sensitivity to motion or visual cues, which could exacerbate their vertigo symptoms.

The underlying cause of vertigo might affect the particular combination and severity of symptoms. For a correct diagnosis, it's critical that people with severe or recurrent vertigo get medical attention. An expert in healthcare can perform a comprehensive assessment, which might involve imaging tests, to determine the reason and create a suitable treatment strategy.

Vertigo Types

Various types of vertigo are distinguished by their underlying causes and characteristics. Peripheral and central vertigo are the two primary varieties.

The most prevalent type of peripheral vertigo is called benign paroxysmal positional vertigo (BPPV), which is brought on by head movements like turning over in bed or gazing up. It is frequently linked to sudden, severe vertigo attacks.

Meniere's disease is characterized by recurrent episodes of vertigo, tinnitus (ear ringing), hearing loss, and a pressured or full sensation in the affected ear.

Vestibular Neuritis: Caused by inflammation of the vestibular nerve, this condition results in abrupt dizziness that is frequently accompanied by nausea and unsteadiness.

Labyrinthitis: An inner ear inflammation that can result in dizziness, hearing loss, and occasionally ringing in the ears.

Vertigo in the center:

Vertigo, a symptom of migraines, can also include headache, light sensitivity, and other migraine symptoms. This condition is known as vestibular migraine.

Brainstem or Cerebellar Disorders: Tumors, strokes, multiple sclerosis, and other conditions affecting the brainstem or cerebellum can result in central vertigo.

Vertebrobasilar Insufficiency: Vertigo is frequently brought on by head movements and is caused by decreased blood supply to the rear of the brain.

Vertigo caused by psychosis:

Anxiety and panic disorders are examples of psychological conditions that can aggravate vertigo and dizziness symptoms.

Vertigo in Position:

Positional vertigo is the term for the vertigo that some people experience solely when they are in particular head postures. One typical case of positional vertigo is BPPV.

Vertigo in rotation:

This kind of vertigo is characterized by a spinning or rotating feeling that is frequently brought on by adjustments to head position or movement.

General Lightheadedness:

Some people may feel lightheaded all the time without experiencing a distinct spinning feeling. There are a number of possible causes for this generalized dizziness, such as medicines or dehydration.

Determining the type of vertigo is essential for a precise diagnosis and suitable management. To identify the precise cause of vertigo, a medical practitioner, such as an otolaryngologist or neurologist, can do a comprehensive evaluation that may involve a medical history, physical examination, and diagnostic tests.

CHAPTER TWO

Identification

When diagnosing vertigo, medical professionals conduct a thorough evaluation to find the underlying cause and formulate a suitable treatment strategy. The following could be a part of the diagnosis process:

Health Background:

The patient's medical history, including information regarding the beginning, length, and features of vertigo episodes, will be gathered by healthcare professionals. We'll talk about any related symptoms, prescriptions, and past health issues.

Physical Assessment:

A comprehensive physical examination will be performed, emphasizing evaluation of eye movements, balance, and coordination. Healthcare professionals may carry out particular actions to induce dizziness and watch for any unusual eye movements (nystagmus).

Examining the nervous system:

To evaluate how well the nervous system which includes the brain and the nerves involved in balance and coordination is working, a neurological examination is essential.

Dix-Hallpike Strategy:

The diagnosis of benign paroxysmal positional vertigo (BPPV) is frequently made with this procedure. It entails putting the person in particular positions to induce vertigo, which aids in determining which ear is injured.

Testing with audiometry:

To evaluate hearing function, hearing tests like audiometry can be performed, particularly in situations of vertigo linked to hearing loss (such Meniere's illness).

Tests of Vestibular Function:

Electronystagmography (ENG) and the caloric test are two tests that evaluate vestibular function and can be used to detect anomalies in the inner ear.

Imaging Research:

To rule out malignancies, structural abnormalities, or other brain problems, imaging procedures like computed tomography (CT) scans or magnetic resonance imaging (MRI) may be required in certain situations.

Blood Examinations:

Blood tests can be used to look for autoimmune illnesses, metabolic abnormalities, infections, and other underlying medical conditions.

EEG (Electroencephalogram):

To evaluate brain activity and rule out causes of vertigo unrelated to seizures, an EEG may be carried out.

Testing with Tilt Tables:

Orthostatic hypotension and other disorders associated with alterations in posture can be assessed with tilt table testing.

Depending on the hypothesized cause of vertigo based on the patient's symptoms and examination results, a specific diagnostic strategy will be used. For an accurate diagnosis and suitable treatment, people with severe or recurrent vertigo must seek medical help as soon as possible.

Strategies for Treatment

The underlying cause of vertigo determines the best course of treatment. The following are typical methods for treating vertigo:

Therapy for vestibular rehabilitation (VRT):

VRT is a kind of physical therapy used to lessen vertigo symptoms and enhance balance. It entails particular workouts designed to improve adaptability and target the vestibular system.

Canalith Maneuvers of Repositioning:

The Epley maneuver is one of these techniques that works well for benign paroxysmal positional vertigo (BPPV). They entail a sequence of head and torso movements intended to realign the inner ear's dislodged calcium crystals.

Drugs:

Medication prescriptions may be issued in response to the underlying cause. As examples, consider:

Antihistamines: Used to treat motion sickness symptoms.

Antiemetics: Drugs that prevent vomiting and nausea.

Benzodiazepines: These drugs may occasionally be administered to treat vertigo-related anxiety.

Vestibular suppressants: Drugs that, in order to reduce symptoms, inhibit the vestibular system.

Handling of Concomitant Disorders:

It is essential to address the underlying cause. Vertigo can be lessened by, for instance, treating infections, treating Meniere's disease with food modifications and medication, or managing migraines.

Modifications to Diet and Lifestyle:

It can be advantageous to make dietary and lifestyle changes. For example, cutting back on salt may help control Meniere's disease symptoms.

Drinking plenty of water

Being well hydrated is crucial since dehydration can exacerbate vertigo and dizziness.

Handling Stress:

Vertigo can be controlled with the use of stress-reduction tactics including mindfulness training and relaxation exercises, particularly if stress aggravates symptoms.

Surgical Procedures:

Surgical procedures might be considered in several situations. For example, surgery to address structural defects in the inner ear or decompress the vestibular nerve.

Drugs Used to Treat Vestibular Migraines:

Prescription drugs for migraine prophylaxis may be necessary if vertigo is a symptom of a migraine.

Support and Guidance:

Counseling and psychological assistance may be helpful, particularly for those who are experiencing worry or emotional discomfort along with vertigo.

For an accurate diagnosis and suitable treatment plan, people with persistent or recurrent vertigo should get evaluated by a medical professional. A multidisciplinary approach combining medical specialists like neurologists, otolaryngologists, and physical therapists may be advised, and treatment may be customized to address the unique cause of vertigo.

Modifications to Lifestyle

Modifying one's lifestyle can assist control and lessen the effects of vertigo. Even though the underlying cause of vertigo may not be cured, these adjustments can enhance general health and the quality of life for those who experience it. The following lifestyle modifications:

Dietary Adjustments:

Low-Sodium Diet: Cutting back on salt can assist control inner ear fluid balance and relieve symptoms in people with illnesses like Meniere's disease.

Drinking plenty of water

It's critical to stay properly hydrated to avoid dehydration, which can exacerbate vertigo.

Steer clear of triggers:

Determine which causes can exacerbate vertigo episodes and stay away from them. This could apply to specific meals, drinks, or pastimes.

Frequent Workout:

Regularly performing mild exercise can help lower stress and enhance general health.

Exercises like yoga, swimming, and walking could be helpful. People should, however, refrain from engaging in activities that cause or exacerbate vertigo.

Sufficient Sleep:

A healthy sleep schedule is essential for general wellbeing. Better sleep can be achieved by establishing a regular sleep schedule and designing a cozy sleeping space.

Handling Stress:

Vertigo symptoms might be made worse by stress. It can be helpful to engage in stress-reduction practices like deep breathing, mindfulness, or meditation.

Avert Coffee and Alcohol:

Caffeine and alcohol can interfere with the vestibular system and make vertigo symptoms worse. It could be advised to limit or stay away from certain substances.

Fall Safety:

Take precautions to avoid falling, particularly when experiencing dizziness. This can entail installing handrails, getting rid of trip hazards, and making sure there is enough lighting.

Helping Tools:

Utilizing assistive technology, such walkers or canes, can occasionally offer stability and support while lowering the chance of falling.

CHAPTER THREE

Frequent medical examinations:

It's critical to schedule follow-up visits with medical professionals on a regular basis to assess any changes in symptoms, modify treatment regimens, and monitor the condition.

Body-Mind Techniques:

Activities that combine mindfulness and soft movements, like tai chi or qi gong, can aid with stress management and balance improvement.

It's critical that people with vertigo collaborate closely with medical professionals to identify the best lifestyle modifications for their particular illness. Combining these modifications with medical procedures and therapies can help manage vertigo holistically and enhance general quality of life.

Handling Dizziness

Self-care, self-support, and practical strategies are all part of managing vertigo. The following coping strategies will help you deal with vertigo:

Learn for Yourself:

Find out more about the causes, symptoms, and possible treatments for the particular kind of vertigo you experience. Gaining knowledge about the illness might enable you to take charge and make wise choices.

Observe treatment schedules:

Follow the recommended course of treatment as directed by your physician. The secret to controlling vertigo symptoms is constancy, whether it comes from prescription drugs, physical therapy, or lifestyle modifications.

Perform these exercises for vestibular rehabilitation:

Participate in vestibular rehabilitation activities that a physical therapist has prescribed. These exercises can lessen the frequency and severity of vertigo episodes in addition to helping with balance.

Safety Measures:

Take steps to reduce the possibility of falling when experiencing episodes of vertigo. Employ handrails, eliminate trip risks from your home, and, if required, think about employing assistive technology.

Determine Triggers:

To find out what causes vertigo attacks to get worse, keep a notebook. Identifying and avoiding these triggers can aid in the management of symptoms.

Control Your Stress:

Vertigo symptoms might be made worse by stress. Include stress-relieving activities in your everyday routine, such as yoga, meditation, or deep breathing.

Maintain Hydration:

Remain properly hydrated because being dehydrated can make you feel lightheaded. Water should be consumed in moderation throughout the day.

Create a Schedule:

Create a daily schedule that consists of regular eating, sleeping, and activity times. Stability can be enhanced by consistency.

Get Emotional Assistance:

Talk about your experiences with loved ones, friends, or support networks. Understanding and emotional support can be obtained by having a support network.

Think about counseling:

Consider getting counseling or therapy if your emotional health is significantly impacted by vertigo in order to manage any tension or anxiety the disease may cause.

Remain Active While Respecting Boundaries:

Take part in physical activities that you feel comfortable and safe doing. Walking and swimming are examples of gentle exercises that can improve general wellbeing.

Employ Calming Methods:

To reduce tension and foster calm, use relaxation methods like progressive muscle relaxation or guided visualization.

Make a Detailed Episode Plan:

Plan ahead and be prepared for periods of vertigo. During episodes, make sure you're in a secure and encouraging setting.

Remain Up to Date:

Keep up with the latest advancements in vertigo treatment. Your healthcare professional should be consulted about any worries or inquiries.

Vertigo management is a unique experience that may need for a mix of coping mechanisms in order to effectively control symptoms and enhance day-to-day functioning. Effective management of vertigo necessitates proactive self-care, emotional support, and regular communication with healthcare experts.

In summary, vertigo is a complicated and frequently difficult condition marked by a mistaken feeling of spinning or lightheadedness. It can have a major effect on a person's everyday functioning by impairing their coordination, balance, and general well-being. Even while vertigo is not a disease in and of itself, it is important for those who experience it to understand its causes, symptoms, and therapy options.

Even though vertigo can be difficult to manage, there is hope for better quality of life and improved management because to advances in medical knowledge and treatment alternatives. For those managing the intricacies of vertigo, seeking prompt medical assistance, remaining informed, and taking a proactive approach to lifestyle management all contribute to a more optimistic view.

THE END